12 Tips for Growing Longer Hair and Retaining Length

Yolanda Victoria

DEDICATION

This book is dedicated to those that believed in me and have always had my back no matter how crazy my plans or dreams may have been. To my sisters, Kenya and Jess, you ladies inspire me every day and I love you both more than you may ever know. Thanks for reminding me everyday in the group chat that my poop does stank! I try every day to be the best big sister I can be and to lead by example. Always follow your dreams and let no one steer you from them. Hey Kayson and Savon, auntie loves you!

To momma, I am so beyond happy with how our relationship continues to blossom every single day. I appreciate every thing you have done for us! Jak wouldn't be the little person that he is today without your guidance and help with EVERY THING. We love you forever.

To daddy, I remember the conversation we had when I first told you that I wanted to become a hairstylist. Every one told me every negative thing they could about becoming a hair stylist but it was you that sat me on the curb in front of the house and said, "follow your heart. You can become the next Vidal Sassoon if you want to. Don't let anyone tell what you can and cannot do." For that much needed push, I can never repay you.

To all of my Jays, you guys are my main motivation and I love you guys! Jak you are the best toddler ever and mommy loves you! Finally, to all of my client over the years, thank you for entrusting me with your hair!

CONTENTS

Yolanda Victoria

What should you expect to know after reading this book?

- Why you should take advice from the author of this ebook.
- This mini book is meant to be a basic format for many of those that are struggling with hair growth and retaining length due to dryness or simply not knowing where to start.
- How to retain length.
- How to encourage hair growth.
- Some of my favorite products.
- The importance of keeping your hair moisturized.
- How to avoid frustrations when trying to achieve your hair length goals.
- The tips provided in this book are not listed in order of importance – they are all equally important.

1 INTRODUCTION

Hi! Thank you for your purchase. My name is Yolanda Victoria, and I have been a healthy hair stylist for close to 20 years and the owner of Gorgeous Strands and Makeup, LLC since 2010. I, personally, have been natural for 17 years on and off. My hair at its longest was four inches below my bra strap (when straightened). I have always experimented with new products and techniques with my hair over the course of two decades and during that time I experienced a lot of setbacks as well as major breakthroughs, but most importantly, I learned some consistent patterns that all hair types need!

Being in the beauty industry for so long, and working with all textures of hair from 1a-4z, has taught me a thing or two about the personality of hair and how to speak the language of hair growth. I am sharing with you some of the things that I have learned over the years!

If my tips are followed, the results will come. I have helped clients over the years achieve growth that they never thought was possible.

2 KNOWING YOUR HAIR TYPE, DENSITY AND POROSITY

Before starting any hair regime, it is very important to know your hair type, hair density, and hair porosity. Knowing these will help you choose the proper products for your hair and help you to avoid purchasing unnecessary products that you cannot use.

The term *hair type* can be described as your hair's curl pattern or lack thereof. There are four types of hair. Type one usually is straight with very little to no curl. Think Jennifer Aniston. Type two is hair that has loose body waves. Think Jennifer Lopez. Type three hair has smaller deep waves. Think Tracee Ellis-Ross. Lastly, type four hair is coiled hair. Think Teyonah Parris. All four types have different wave, curls or coil size variations within that group type.

Hair density is how thick or thin your hair is on the whole head and how closely placed your hair strands are on the scalp. The more strands per square inch you have, the thicker (or more dense) your hair is. For instance, if you can easily see your scalp when styling your hair, you more than likely have less dense hair. If your hair strands are very close together and you can barely see your scalp, you have thick density. A person can also have medium density meaning the hair falls in between less dense and most dense.

Note: Two people can have the same hair type but have different density. Two people can also have different hair types and the same density.

Hair porosity is the ability of the hair to absorb moisture or products. There are three types of hair porosity low, normal, and high.

Low porosity hair allows for very little moisture to penetrate the hair. If you feel like hair products sit on top of your hair and do not absorb, you likely have low porosity. You can also tell low porosity hair by noticing at the end of the day, no matter how much moisture you use, the hair still is very dry.

Normal porosity hair typically holds in moisture and allows for product to penetrate the hair shaft. Normal porosity hair rarely struggles with dryness or hair not maintaining its moisture throughout the day.

High porosity hair is typically chemically treated hair that soaks in too much product instantly but loses the moisture just as quickly.

3 TRIMMING YOUR ENDS

While trimming your hair on the ends will not ensure that your hair grows from the scalp, trimming off dead ends will ensure you retain length and keep split ends from spreading. Trimming too much can affect length as well. If you are trimming every six weeks, you are trimming too much in order to retain length. If you are already experiencing problems growing or retaining length, the last thing you should be doing is trimming or cutting your hair too often.

When length retention is the goal a good time frame, on average, is to have the ends trimmed quarterly if you wear hair styles that require a lot manipulation (flat ironing, blow drying, etc.). If you wear low manipulation styles (wash and go, twist or braid outs, etc.) then a good end trim two-three times a year will suffice. Over-trimming can also lead to the false belief that your hair has gotten to a certain length and stopped growing or your hair is in a "growth halt."

Please keep in mind that if you trim your own ends and decide against going to a professional do not, I repeat, do not use the same shears you use to cut weave tracks, paper, meat or any other household misc. items. Using the wrong shears can lead to trimming your ends with dull shears which causes split ends. Imagine this, you trimmed your ends to get rid of split ends, and you added split ends with dull shears—that's completely counter-productive. Trimming with dull shears has now led to shorter hair with new split ends. Please invest in a pair of shears that is strictly for trimming hair ends.

If you do go to a professional, make sure the professional is well versed in trimmed/cutting curly and/or textured hair. Do not assume just because the person is a hair stylist that he or she should know how to trim or cut your curly hair. All hair stylists are not created equally. A little research will save you a lot of headache.

It is also important to note that the hair does not need to be straightened to have curly ends trimmed or cut.

4 COMBING/BRUSHING

Some people are against brushing or combing, but when done right you will have greater control over the hair and less tangling. Starting with very small sections brush or comb your hair beginning with the ends and working your way up the strands. Working your way up the strands, in small sections, decreases unnecessary breakage caused by manipulation like brushing or combing. Never brush your hair while dry. Always use a large toothed detangling comb and never a small tooth comb.

Brushing your hair while the product (conditioner, moisturizer, leave in, etc.) is in your hair ensures the product is evenly disturbed throughout and all strands are moisturized equally. Evenly distributed product creates a properly moisturized head of hair. By now, we all know the importance of moisture and how it relates to length retention. Brushing also encourages curl clumping.

Curl clumping = #hairgoals

My favorite brush is all black Denman Brush with 9 rows.

5 COVER UP YOUR HAIR

At bedtime, whether your hair is styled or not, make sure your hair is properly tied up in a scarf, bonnet, or sleep on a satin or t-shirt covered pillow to prevent the hair from drying out or tangling overnight. Drying out your hair promotes breakage and split ends. As we know the goal in length retention is to keep the hair as moisturized as possible and to protect the ends as much as possible, including when it is time for sleep. Not covering your hair at night resets all of the moisturizing you have been consistently doing with you hair throughout the week. One time of not covering the hair during bedtime can remove days' worth of moisture.

Covering your hair while in the shower is as equally important as covering while asleep. If you want to maintain a style, it is advisable to use a plastic or non-porous shower cap during your showers.

Covering your hair during showers eliminates unnecessary manipulation and allowing you to maintain a style much longer. Covering your hair and protecting your style in the shower is not to be confused with intentionally wetting or cleansing your hair in the shower.

Your local beauty supply store has some great and inexpensive shower caps and bonnets that stay on throughout the showers and overnight!

6 WET YOUR HAIR AND DRINK YOUR WATER

I tell my clients all the time "treat your hair like your favorite plant." One of the main things that plants survive off of is consistent watering – same with your hair. Just as water nourishes the inside of your body, it works the same on the outside. Water is an excellent source of moisture for the hair. Take advantage! Once I started to wet my hair regularly during the week, I started to experience lots of growth, and my hair became stronger than ever! Part of the reason that a lot of people do not experience the ultimate growth is due to misinformation such as "black people should not wet their all the time." Not only is this information false but it has made a lot of African Americans fearful of getting our hair which has led us to not want to swim, workout or just enjoy without worrying about messing up a hair style!

Water on the hair promotes length retention and hair growth! And, do not forget to drink up!

7 SUPPLEMENTS, DERMATOLOGY AND HORMONES

While hair products work on the outside, hair supplements work on the inside! Achieving maximum hair growth requires work on the in and outside of the bodies so proper nutrition is key!

Maintaining a healthy nutrient-rich diet is not always easy for some. To ensure your body has the proper nourishment to release healthy hair take some form of healthy hair vitamin. GNC Women's Advanced Hair, Skin and Nail Formula work well! GNC has been a leading and trusted supplement provider for decades and are slightly less expensive than some of the more recent, popular hair vitamins on the market. This supplement contains key hair growth inducing vitamins such as biotin and b-6 to help you on your hair growth journey.

It is important to keep in mind that some supplements will work better for others. For example, if you are one that does not normally consume healthy foods that contain proper nutrients for your hair and you start to take supplements you may see greater results than someone that eat healthy and consume water on a regular basis. This is not to suggest that those that eat healthy should not think of taking a daily supplement, the example was provided to show that your results may vary.

It is important to do your research on the supplement you decide to take before consuming. Also, please consult your doctor before consuming any vitamins.

If you have been taking a supplement consistently for six months without change and If you feel like you have done every thing in your power to achieve healthy hair yet you are still facing hair brittleness and breakage it is definitely time to consult with your physician. Sometimes no matter how healthy of a hair care routine you have the underlining issue may be something below the skin that cannot be treated topically. After suffering the effects of imbalanced hormones personally I can tell you for sure getting a full female hormonal panel is an extremely important step to take; not just for your hair but overall healthiness. As females, our hormones can wreak havoc on our bodies and hair is typically one of the first signs that hormones may be out of balanced.

I can proudly say that whether relaxed or natural I have been able to maintain a healthy full head of hair, taken some form of hair vitamins, kept my hair cleansing and conditioning routine on point and have kept a pretty good, not great, diet. Needless to say it came as a shocker to me when I started experiencing brittle and breaking hair. I had no idea what had changed. At the time, I was natural and had no chemicals in my hair. I was still on the same hair regime, still working out, drinking water and just overall pridefully caring for the hair that I had loved so much over the years. I truly thought it was something that was in my hair cabinet and ditched everything and started anew, only to still have extremely dry, brittle and breaking hair. Soon realizing the damage was not triggered by something that I was using on my hair topically I went to Dr. Google and started doing my research on potential causes of unexplained hair loss and was lead to my hormones. I quickly made an appointment with my OB/Gyn and requested a full hormone panel (FHP). After getting a FHP done I found out that I was very deficient in Vitamin D, along with some other imbalances that could have also contributed to my unexpected hair loss. Vitamin D deficiencies can lead to hair loss. My research on vitamin d and hair loss began. I followed the instructions of my OB/GYN and took my high dose of Vitamin D daily for six weeks. After the course of about three months I did notice a difference in the feel of my hair. At that point, however, the damage was done. I was glad to find out the cause of damage but I was not feeling my new look at all.

I had enough with looking at my hair and decided one day to cut it off at the breaking point and started over. That was in August 2013. For a little over a year I wore protective styles. I still focused on moisturizing my hair during these protective, as I knew protective styles were not going to be permanent and the ultimate goal was for me to wear my healthy hair again. By late 2014 my hair was back to armpit length, full and shiny! I then decided to ditch the protective styles and get back to my hair. I was so happy!

If you have gotten your hormones all checked out and everything looks great but you are still having hair issues then it may be time for a visit to the dermatologist. Scalp disorders can come in all forms and most times these disorders are not visible to the naked eye. A visit to your dermatologist can lead you on the right path to treating hair that seems to grow at an extremely slow rate or simply not grow at all. Scalp funguses, tension alopecia, scalp psoriasis and eczema can be discovered and treated by a dermatologist. It is important to note that you should find a dermatologist that has worked on and successfully treated hair issues that you are struggling with.

8 CONDITION! CONDITION! CONDITION!

Conditioning may seem like a no-brainer to some but as a hair stylist of 18 years, using a conditioning treatment is not high on the priority list for a lot of clients that have sat in my hair. Most people truly believe you can get away with conditioning your hair only when visiting a professional or just skipping conditioner altogether is fine. This misinformation is completely false. The hair requires a good deep conditioning weekly in order to perform at its best.

If you do not focus on ANY other product ever in life make sure you focus on a conditioner that works well for your hair. The right conditioner is the hairs best friend, hands down. Not shampoo, conditioner. Shampoo cleanses and does not necessarily promotes growth or strengthen the hair. Conditioner, however, promotes growth AND strength of the hair. The benefits of regularly conditioning your hair are endless including providing softness and manageability. Conditioners also provide a good slip on the hair to make combing or brushing out easier, which decreases the likely hood of unnecessary hair breakage.

The reason lots of time people are unable to retain length is due to not have a proper conditioner or conditioning routine. Not using a conditioner on a regular basis leads to dryness. Dryness leads to breakage. Breakage means you are not retaining length. Not retaining length makes you think your hair is not growing.

In order to avoid dry ends make sure you start your hair week off with a great deep conditioning product. Apply a liberal amount of conditioner to your ends first and work your way up the strand to the roots. Using this method ensures all hairs are being conditioned.

9 KEEP SCALP CLEAR OF PRODUCT BUILDUP

With all of the co-washing (cleansing the hair with conditioner instead of shampoo), pre-pooing (prepping the hair with moisture before shampooing), product overload and avoiding shampoos, product buildup is inevitable. Prolonged product buildup can lead to clogged pores on your scalp. Keep scalp follicles clear to allow the sebum to flow and healthy hair to grow in. (Sebum is the scalps natural oils)

While we are on the subject of cleansing, it is important to know that shampooing the hair too much can also cause dryness. Shampoos have certain ingredients that are made to cleanse the hair, but in turn, those same ingredients strip the hair of its natural moisture. Some of those main ingredients that help cleanse the hair but strip the hair of its natural oils are detergents known as Ammonium Laurel Sulfate and Sodium Lauryl Sulfate (SLS). Simply put shampooing your curly hair even weekly can be too drying, especially if you already have dry hair and are using the wrong shampoo for our hair type.

If you typically like to style your hair weekly then bi-weekly shampooing your hair is fine in conjunction with weekly co-washes.

10 PROMOTE INCREASED BLOOD CIRCULATION TO THE SCALP

Did you know increased blood circulation to the scalp promotes faster hair growth? The reason people hair seem to grow faster than others is because of the amount of blood circulation (and natural oils) leading to the scalp. Have you noticed that your scalp feels tight and dry and your friend's hair, who grows long, scalp seems loose, soft and pliable? Tight scalp typically doesn't get the proper amount of blood circulation or natural oils coming to the scalp and may need a little jumpstart. Achieving soft, pliable and moisturized scalp and hair is the key to promoting healthy, speedy hair growth.

Some things you can do to promote increased blood circulation to the scalp area are nightly scalp massages, hair steaming and your favorite cardio exercise – Zumba anyone?!

My Favorite: I give my scalp a light massage while I am in the shower. The steam and massage promote blood circulation!

11 MOISTURIZING – LOC, LCO AND LOCO

One common complaint I hear about curly hair is dryness. People with straight hair want to stay away from oiliness as much as possible whereas the curly girls want to keep the hair moisturized as much as possible. Why is it that people with straight always seem to have moisturized/oily hair? The natural oils can travel down straight hair with ease. There are no s-shaped waves, coils or curls for the oil to travel down, just a straight highway for the oil to travel with ease. Oil had a rollercoaster of a ride to take with curly hair. Somewhere along the curl the oil stops and leaves the ends thirsty! Thirsty ends is the main reason moisturizing the hair is so necessary.

Now that we know a little more about why curly hair gets dry easily let's discuss the different ways to moisturize the hair. If you are unfamiliar with the letters (LOC, LCO, LOCO) in the chapter name and have hair that struggles to retain moisture, then this chapter is definitely for you! When speaking to clients about their dry hair, I have realized that most clients use the LOC, the most popular method, without knowing there are other methods of sealing oil into your hair. If you have tried the LOC method and it did not try one of the other methods!

For those of you that do not know the meaning of LOC, LCO, LOCO, here is the breakdown:

L = Liquid or Leave-in (must be water based).

O = Oil. Keep in mind the different types of oils. Thicker oils are for dense hard to penetrate hair, and thinner/lighter oils are for finer easier to penetrate hair.

C = cream. Your favorite styling cream can be used.

L(iquid)CO method is good for normal to medium density hair types 3c/4a/4b that can use some moisture but already has some good clump to the curls.

L(eave in cream)OC method is good for clients with denser and thicker hair types 4b/4c.

LOCO. This step is basically the LOC method with the oil as the finishing sealant. Typically those with super thirsty hair that does not stay moisturized looking throughout the day can benefit from the LOCO method.

Implementing one of these methods into your hair regimen will increase the moisture level which will make the hair easier to manage, comb and help prevent breakage when styling. Keep in mind your hair type and density when using any of these methods. If your hair is fine and dry putting too much product will weigh it down where as if your hair is dense and dry putting too little product will leave the hair dry.

12 PROTECTIVE STYLES

Protective styles are necessary to give the hair a break from over manipulation. When frustration starts to rear its ugly little head, clients tend to take out the frustration on their hair. Frustrations lead to pulling and tugging harder than normal which lead to unnecessary breakage. Or the hair is simply neglected.

Protective styling allows our hair to just be and grow at its own pace without being bothered.

Have you ever met someone with long, amazing hair and you ask her what she does to it and she says, "nothing, really." What you are witnessing is protective styling at its finest. Leaving the hair alone can be a good thing when done right. If the more you comb, the more hair you see on the floor or in the sink means the more you probably need to step back and give you and your hair a rest. Some protective styling options are: cornrows, individual braids (not too tight on the edges) sew ins without leave out and natural hair up-dos like twists.

While you are wearing a protective, you still should spray a liquid leave in on the hair and keep your hair and scalp oiled. A lot of times it is easy to forget that the hair still needs to be moisturized while in protective styles. Be mindful of how the style starts to look. If your style starts to look dry, moisturize it. Keeping your hair moisturized while in a protective style allows you to transition back to your natural hair without having to put in extra work to get the hairs moisture levels back to normal.

Finally, a protective style is not a protective style if you lose your edges in the process. Please do not choose a style that will do unnecessary permanent damage to your edges – no style is ever worth losing your edges.

My favorite protective style: Custom wigs. With wigs, I can take them off whenever I want so I can give my hair and scalp some much needed tender love and care!

13 STAY CONSISTENT

Consistency is probably one of the most important steps that people may forget about. This process is not always easy or fun but staying the course will be greatly rewarding and empowering!

One way to stay consistent is to come up with a hair plan. A hair plan is very similar to meal-planning. In meal planning, you plan and prepare your menu and meals weekly so you can avoid frustration and eating something that you should not be eating. With the hair plan you will create a list of styles you will do on your hair, get your products stocked up, choose your prep night and wash day, and finally, choose wrapping or tying up methods nightly that will keep your styles fresh throughout the week.

Find brands of hair products that work for your hair and stick to them. Only change if you start to notice the products do not work well with your hair anymore. This is not the time to experiment with your hair because experimenting leads to frustrations and doing something to your hair that you may regret in the long run if you do not get your desired hair goals.

For now, stick to basic products – cleanser, conditioner, oil, leave in, styling cream. Add products after you feel you have mastered your current lineup of products or a product isn't blending well with other products.

Keep your hair goals in mind by creating a vision board. Again, frustrations creep in and make you lose your focus, and a vision board will be a friendly reminder of what you are trying to achieve with your hair. Have the vision board where you normally do your hair regime, on your screen saver at work, your home screen on your phone and anywhere else that you frequent. The vision of your hair goals helps to avoid cutting or relaxing the hair when you do not know what else to do.

Following these tips consistently will help you throughout your journey and help you achieve growth that you have always wanted. Do not forget to follow me on social media and show me your progress. Use the tag #12tipstohairgrowth so I can see them! I believe in you!

COPYRIGHT

First Printing: 2017

ISBN <978-1-387-03236-5>

Gorgeous Strands and Makeup, LLC

PO BOX 773347

Houston, TX 77215

For regular hair tips and updates follow me on Instagram, Facebook and Twitter @gorgeousstrands

www.gorgeousstrands.com

www.ingramcontent.com/pod-product-compliance
Lightning Source LLC
Chambersburg PA
CBHW050352290526
45785CB00006B/2734